What Your Doctor Won't Tell You About Weight Loss

What Your Doctor Won't Tell You About Weight Loss

✦

Mesotherapy and More

Dr. Roberta Foss-Morgan

iUniverse, Inc.

New York Lincoln Shanghai

What Your Doctor Won't Tell You About Weight Loss
Mesotherapy and More

iUniverse, Inc.

For information address:
iUniverse, Inc.
2021 Pine Lake Road, Suite 100
Lincoln, NE 68512
www.iuniverse.com

ISBN: 0-595-32229-8

Printed in the United States of America

Contents

G

INTRODUCTION

I am an anti-aging physician. Anti-aging physicians have acquired an MD or a DO degree and have chosen to practice medicine in an integrative way. Anti-aging medicine is a marriage between conventional MD allopathic training and complementary medicine.

Another way to describe the type of medicine I do is internal plastic surgery. Many plastic surgeons I have met explain that to have a good result outside, you need treatment on the inside. Using methods I learned from European endocrinologists, I have found effective ways of treating the inside. I deal with a number of maladies, from Chronic Fatigue Syndrome and Fibromyalgia, to Attention Deficit Disorder and Immune Enhancement post-chemotherapy. I treat with biochemically-identical, or non-synthetic, hormone replacement therapy, a method I learned from European endocrinologists. I also treat patients who desire to lose weight. Because excess weight will eventually manifest itself as Hypertension, Coronary Artery Disease, Cancer, etc., it's important to deal with it before it becomes a larger problem.

I do not practice alternative medicine, which very often does not require a medical degree. Practicing anti-aging medicine requires thousands upon thousands of hours of further training, and traveling throughout the United States, as well as Europe, to learn prevention and reversal of chronic degenerative diseases.

Learning about medicine, nutrition, exercise, and reversing chronic degenerative disease is my hobby, as well as my job. I am a rigorous scholar who loves to learn. Learning for me is fun. I am passionately curious about everything, especially how I can help patients remain well. Einstein said, "We live in a world of problems which can no longer be solved by the level of thinking which created them." This is why I am so enamored by integrative medicine. It requires me to think creatively and differently than the way I was taught.

Integrative physicians embrace our conventional training, even prescribing FDA-approved pharmaceuticals when necessary. We are different from conventional medicine, however, because we don't stop there. Integrative physicians do what works, read international medical studies, and remember that the goal is to do no harm to patients. In my mind, practicing medicine with a prescription pad may help me feel as though I am doing what I have been trained to do, but I know that prescribing medication for every ailment that patients report may hurt them more than help them.

Practicing medicine this way requires becoming comfortable with chaos, constant study, and a brain willing to be flexible and change. Unlike other physicians, I reach out to my patients to have them teach me, instead of just teaching them. They bring me books, Internet research, and medical articles. I often say my higher power brings what I need to learn, relearn, and over-learn via my patients. And this is how I came to learn about Mesotherapy.

During a routine follow-up consultation for biochemically-identical hormone replacement therapy, a patient asked me if I knew about Mesotherapy. I had seen the word once or twice, but wasn't entirely sure what it meant. I researched it, and found the only place to be trained in Mesotherapy is Paris. Eager to study and understand this new weight loss technique, I boarded a plane to France.

I discovered, among many other things, that Mesotherapy is actually not new. It has been done in Europe for five decades to dissolve fat in those places that are resistant to fat loss, no matter how much exercise and dietary control we employ. It is a safer and healthier alternative to liposuction surgery, previously the only option available in the United States.

Upon arrival home, I wondered if Mesotherapy really worked. I only saw and treated each patient one time, not having the luxury of observing follow-up results. I performed Mesotherapy on myself, and after one treatment, my pants were loose, and my baggy knees were looking pretty perky.

I quickly realized, however, that Mesotherapy is just a jumpstart for those who are already involved in their present and future healthcare, and want to be healthier and leaner. Our practice policy is to only accept patients who are strength training twice a week, who know the difference between complex and refined carbohydrates, and who partake in adequate daily protein. In short, we only accept Mesotherapy patients who are not only interested in losing weight, but who are also interested in staying healthy.

Mesotherapy is not for morbidly obese patients. It is also not for patients who have had gastric bypass surgery, and are not at the point where they can do strength training. Mesotherapy is not an immediate answer; it will only aid you in your quest to de-fat those problematic areas resistant to exercise and whole food nutrition.

We can lose a little over one pound of fat per week. Those commercials telling you that you can lose ten pounds of fat per week are fooling you. You can lose water, and, more importantly, muscle by dieting. In fact, with each week spent immobile, you lose 0.9% of muscle per week. You will end up in worse shape than before you started. In order for Mesotherapy to work, and, more importantly, to stay healthy, you need to understand what you do 21 times a week: eat.

Aside from the fact that fat easily makes you look ten to fifteen years older, fat also contains toxins. During the Arizona Biosphere experiment, people lost fat too quickly when they lived in a controlled environment. There were no toxins because they were in a clean, non-chemicalized environment, and they ate totally organic foods. As they lost weight the stored toxins in their fat made them feel unwell. This is called the Herxheimer Reaction. As you release toxins and metabolic breakdown products, you actually feel worse before you feel better.

Releasing those toxins from your body is the first step to losing weight, as well as achieving longevity. Living to 100 years old and beyond is futile unless we have accompanying function. To do this, you not only need to understand what to eat, but also why certain foods are better for you than others, how the way you eat affects your body, and why physicians are not properly trained in nutrition. You must be willing to open your mind, and unlearn things you were previously taught were law. This change will come slowly, piece by piece, like a puzzle.

Let's learn, change, and think together. We'll begin with understanding the obesity epidemic in America; what caused it, and how we can stop it.

1

The Obesity Epidemic in the US

We are all painfully aware that America has an obesity epidemic. Sixty-four percent of Americans are now overweight, and 31 percent are obese. A person is obese if his or her body-mass index is 30 or above which means a weight about 20 percent over a healthy one. Yearly medical spending on obesity is about 93 billion dollars, and about half of that is paid by Medicare and Medicaid. Obesity is rapidly becoming a trillion dollar disease and will bankrupt our present health cost system.

How did this happen? Why are Americans- who are supposedly so highly educated with plenty of access to whole food nutrition- so overweight? It is astounding that we are the most powerful nation, yet we know so little about how to eat properly. There is very little training in nutrition during our elementary education. Furthermore, there is little to no education in nutritional biochemistry during a doctor's medical training. The obesity epidemic is not completely our fault, but it is important that we learn how and what to eat.

In the US, our portions are gargantuan. A serving of pasta is one-half cup cooked, and restaurants serve three cups—six times the amount required. Add to that an appetizer, bread and butter, drinks, the potato, the salad with croutons (which are the equivalent of two slices of bread), dessert, and maybe after-dinner drinks. A brunch can be 8000 calories. When we go to the movies, popcorn can be well over 2000 calories. Usually people buy soda, and candy, sit for two hours—then go out to eat after the movie. Study after study shows that those who ate 2000 calories at one sitting gained weight, and those who spread the calories throughout the day actually lost weight. As a child, a Coca Cola was six ounces, now we have the sixty-four ounce big gulp. Portions are gargantuan in size because it doesn't cost very much to make your meal the size of your last supper. Many of us were raised with the finish your plate mandate, then you were rewarded with dessert. Is it any wonder we have an obesity epidemic?

Beyond our oversized portions, our lives are moving at a pace that was unheard of even fifty years ago. We are moving so fast, there is no time to slow down and prepare a meal. Many people skip breakfast and wait until they are starving. Others eat only one meal a day, as fast and as voraciously as possible. Even on the rare occasions we get a chance to slow down and enjoy a home-cooked meal, we don't take time to chew thoroughly and digest properly, which can wreak a lot of havoc on our already damaged bodies.

It has been reported that we eat 50% of our meals outside the home, and we eat 15 of our 21 meals at fast food restaurants. Just one lunch at a fast food restaurant can exceed your daily caloric requirements. Because so few of us were taught the most rudimentary elements of nutrition, we don't think about the problems the artificial food we eat so often causes. I am aghast when I peer in a young mother's shopping cart that contains not one single item of real food. While her three children are spinning wildly through the store, she is picking up boxes of sugar-coated cereal and bottles of caffeinated soda. When one mid-western middle school removed the soda and candy machines from it's cafeteria, much of the ADD went away, and the students were more focused and teachable. It was that simple.

It is not just our love of junk food that has caused the obesity epidemic, but also our love of low-fat foods and diets. The fat in low-fat foods has been replaced with four times the sugar, making it no better than the junk food it is an alternative to. Diets cause you to lose water and muscle, which help you break down fat and burn calories. You don't want to lose an ounce of muscle because muscle makes you burn more calories, fat doesn't require calories to remain alive. If you combine dangerous low-fat foods and muscle-reducing diets to restrict calories, your Basal Metabolic Rate (BMR) goes down. This is a survival mechanism inside us that is used to protect our bodies in the event of famine. When you severely restrict the calories, your body doesn't interpret it as healthy weight loss; it interprets it as a crisis.

What we eat- and how we eat- is also connected to our emotional state. In recent years, there have been increasing numbers of gastric bypass surgeries being done in the United States. They take a stomach with a two-quart capacity and reduce it to two ounces. Post-surgery, patients literally shrink before your eyes, many times losing one pound per day. Although this seems to be the Miracle Weight Loss cure some people have been waiting for, there are still many questions to be answered. We are not addressing why these patients ate so much in the first place. Bingeing often represents buried emotional conflict, and food is often used as a tranquilizer, or a substitute for affection. One major reason we crave carbohydrates is because they help our bodies form "feel good" hormones, such as serotonin and dopamine. Our emotional hunger is easily taken care of by carbohydrates. Certain emotions also cause us to store fat, like stress, which increases the fat-storing hormone coritsol. Weight loss requires emotional transformation, as well as physical, so that we can stop this cycle of craving carbs and storing fat.

Now that you have some understanding of the cause of the obesity epidemic in the US, you are probably wondering what can be done to fix it. I believe with religious fervor that the key to reversing the obesity epidemic in America is education. We need more education about nutrition, our bodies, and the toxins in our food. We will never be perfect, but that is not our goal. Our goal is to learn what we need to do to live healthier lives.

This education should begin with an understanding that we are not completely to blame for the obesity epidemic in America. Physicians' medical training in America is somewhat devoid of training in proper nutrition. As important as it is to educate ourselves, it is also important to educate those we trust to ensure our health.

2

Why Doctors Don't Know Enough About Nutrition

Physicians have an interesting way of doing things when they are presented with a paradigm shift. I befriended a Harvard-graduated oncologist who thought the complementary modalities my medical practice added to cancer patients' status post-chemotherapy, radiation, and surgery made perfect sense. However, he refused to take up the practice himself, instead choosing to refer his patients to me. Anything new always goes through three stages: first, it is rejected, then it is recognized for not working, and finally, it's accepted, but with the proviso that they knew it all along.

This has happened with a variety of now-common medical discoveries. Rheumatoid arthritis was considered a psychiatric diagnosis until Cortisone was discovered in the 1920s. It took the ECG 40 years to gain acceptance as the mainstream diagnostic modality for cardiac function. Research on the ability of 400 mcgs of folic acid to prevent Spina Bifida was published 30 years before it's final approval, causing and estimated 250,000 babies to be born with this terrible birth defect. Blood transfusions were done by medical heretics 50 years before they gained acceptance. Now, These are just a sampling of what the mainstream medical community has had trouble accepting in the past. The tradition continues with nutrition, supplementation, and understanding the chronic degenerative diseases of aging. Regardless of the numerous studies and research in support of anti-aging medicines, physicians continue to ignore their possibilities. This is not, however, entirely the physicians' fault. The problem actually begins with a doctor's training in medical school.

During the first three months of medical school, students have over 70 examinations, in a variety of different courses, including histology, emergency medicine, gross anatomy, neurology, physiology, psychiatry, and pharmacology. If you decide to go for a DO degree, you receive five hundred extra hours on spinal manipulation. There is simply not enough time to teach future doctors about nutritional biochemistry, and the importance of prevention and reversal of the chronic degenerative diseases of aging.

As medical training now exists, we are trained to think- and treat patients- in a linear, mechanistic, Newtonian-physics kind of way. If a patient presents with symptoms of an under-active thyroid and the tests agree, the patient is given a prescription and we have done what we were taught. An integrative medical physician has much more to do. What physicians presently do is fix the damage from the leaky roof, but not the leaky roof. Integrative medical physicians fix both. This requires continual learning, and a mind that can think panoramically, embracing both their prescription pad privileges, and whatever else works and does not harm the patient.

How did I end up with in integrative medicine? I was lucky. During the 1970s, while I was training in skating at a national level, I heard the Russians were having their blood tested every Friday, and were taking "supplements". The other American skaters and I were eating the daily fare: hot dogs, hamburgers, soda, and fast food. Something intuitively told me this gave the Russians an advantage.

I happened to pick up a copy of Prevention Magazine, which contained an article describing a state-of-the-art medical facility in Princeton, New Jersey. It was called the Princeton Bio Center. After becoming a patient with the goal to be the strongest athlete I could be, I became very interested in nutritional biochemistry. I read voraciously and attempted to put the puzzle pieces together, but there was so much "doctor-talk", I didn't understand most of what I was reading. I decided to attend medical school to gain a better understanding of it all.

By graduation from my residency, the founder of the Princeton Bio Center passed away, and they needed a Medical Director. I was able to do what I loved, practice medicine and integrate nutrition into the patient's treatment plan. However, there was one problem. The residency program told me that they were very concerned about my accepting this medical directorship. They told me that if I practiced medicine that way, I might very well lose my license. I was surprised at this reaction, but I soon came to understand why they felt that way.

If you think there is peer pressure in high school, you should become a doctor. All doctors want to look, act, and think exactly like their peers. Most physicians are not going to think outside the box until a prestigious medical journal tells them the research has been consistently proven using double-blind studies.

However, there is a problem with this strong belief that something is not proven until it has passed double-blind studies. Because these types of studies are very costly to do, only drug companies have the time and money to do them. It is impossible to patent something that already exists in nature. The drug companies cannot patent antioxidants, CoQl0, or minerals. There is no money to be made doing studies on substances which our bodies make, or which are found in food.

There are literally thousands of studies documenting the mechanism of action and interaction of supplements with medications in order to reverse the chronic degenerative diseases of aging. These studies are primarily found in European medical journals, but are beginning to surface in American medical journals, as well. They show that the herbal supplement Gingko Biloba is the most prescribed substance in Germany, and that all cancer patients in Europe receive prescriptions for mushroom extracts to enhance immune system function. Since most physicians are not aware of these studies, they are not the ones to ask about the benefits of supplementations, or the other topics presented in those studies, like whole food nutrition and natural hormone replacement therapy.

Besides doctors' lack of training and firm belief in double-blind studies, there is also the problem of time. Most physicians simply do not have enough time to spend with you, answering your questions, and teaching you. They would like to, but, as seen in the CNN documentary "Doctors Under the Knife", they spend one third of their day doing paperwork. Some states, like New Jersey, are actually suing the HMOs for practicing medicine without a license. Your physician would truly like to spend hours a day studying to keep up-to-date and teaching their patients, but it's not possible.

Unfortunately, as the medical system now stands, most patients know more about omega 3 fatty acids, pyridoxal 5 phosphate, mineral depletion, and the fact that Tocotrienols are fifty times stronger than Vitamin E than their physician. They get their information from the newest medical journal, the internet. Although patients have a great deal of knowledge, it needs to be tidied up a bit. Since nutritional biochemistry has been my hobby and my career for over three decades now, I am able to answer patients' questions.

That's where this book comes in. Retraining yourself to learn more about becoming healthy and lean is the best investment you can make. Unless you are very fortunate, your physician has not been trained to answer your questions about nutrition and supplements, and how you can regain optimal weight. However, the keys to longevity are within your control. Studies show that those who are happy and healthy take control of their lives early on and never let go. Next, we will talk about a few simple, yet little-known secrets that will help you do just that.

3

9 Simple Weight Loss Tips

Every minute, 7 baby boomers turn 50. However, turning 50 doesn't mean you have to deal with things like memory loss, fatigue, loss of libido, muscle pain, insomnia, gastric reflux, or difficulty losing weight. You can prevent and reverse these symptoms of aging so that, as you get older, you stay functional in all realms. I am 54, and by educating myself on how to stay healthy, I feel better than I did when I was 20, and a national competitor in skating.

Last year I did a little experiment, with myself as the subject. At that time, I had a good 15 pounds of fat to remove. I went to many weight loss centers advertised on television and listened to what they had to say.

The diet plans varied little, usually allowing you about 1, 200 calories per day. However, the calories allowed were chemicalized foods, margarine (which is one molecule short of being plastic), and liberal use of artificial sweeteners. After my diet plan expedition was over, I became acutely aware that even the most well-known weight loss centers didn't know anything about nutritional biochemistry. They were, however, very good at babysitting clients in their quest to become lean. I listened to how people would not lose, or lose for a while and then plateau with their weight loss efforts, and I was passionately curious as to why they were metabolically stuck in their weight loss efforts.

Then, in November of 2002, I attended the Integrative Cancer Conference at Thomas Jefferson University Hospital in Philadelphia. MRIs of tumors were shown, and regardless of where the tumor resided—the liver, pancreas, and colon—I noticed something amazing. The tumors were encased in fat. As the patients went on macrobiotic diets, their subsequent MRIs demonstrated decreased tumor size and simultaneously the fat was disappearing.

I finally understood and accepted what I had been doing wrong. I decided to de-fat my body. I began with a three-day fat fast, eating 250 calories of organic nuts four to five times a day. I did this so I wouldn't lose an ounce of muscle. When I restarted eating on Day Four, I ate one half of what I formerly ate, and I ate it more slowly. I also joined a gym where I prepaid for fifteen personal training sessions, two times a week for one half hour. I only overate when I attended social occasions, parties, barbeques, etc., because weight loss doesn't have to be a totally organic experience 24/7. The results? In 12 short weeks, I lost 15 pounds of fat, 11 pounds on the scale, and gained four pounds of muscle. I quickly followed it up with Mesotherapy, and I needed to buy new slacks two sizes smaller. It was that simple.

In order to attain this type of results in your own journey to lose weight, you must learn what to eat, and how to eat, as well as the benefits of exercise, and how to de-stress.

The French Paradox

The French have a much lower rate of obesity than we do; only 8% obesity compared to 60% in the US. They also eat far more proteins, real dairy, and fats. This is called "The French Paradox". While in Paris, and during the writing of this book, it became less of a paradox to me. I came to the conclusion that, by doing simple things like eating slowly, eating smaller portions, and eating only real foods, anyone can lose weight and keep it off, just as the French do.

The French walk very briskly, everywhere. My medical practice is 1.4 miles from my home. In France, no one would have driven. The expected transportation for that short distance would be a rapid four-mile an hour pace.

The French eat much less sugar than we do. Their major intake of sugar is in the form of wine, taken with their noon and evening meals. Wine- especially red wine- has many healthful components. Drinking wine in moderation has been studied extensively. Those who have never had a drop of alcohol are actually at a health disadvantage according to the studies.

The French also eat and chew slowly, and they do not speak with food in their mouths. They actually dine. They relax, enjoy their meal, and as a result, they end up eating less. This is where I start when counseling a patient for weight control. Eating this way makes us eat about 50% less. Realize, however, that this habit takes a lot of conscious effort.

The French also eat real food, in appropriate portions. I saw no pizza parlors, delicatessens, hoagie shops, or fast food establishments. I did see one McDonalds, which one Parisian told me is new. The French eat large, raw salads with protein, and real cheese. Their dairy is whole fat dairy, which contains a very important component: Conjugated Linoleic Acid (CLA), which is a "good fat" that, among other things, actually helps you lose weight.

The French Paradox has many levels that explain their lower rate of obesity. CLA is a major reason, but all the other lifestyle modalities they do are vitally important as well, including Mesotherapy. As I said before, Mesotherapy is not a procedure that is done every week for the rest of your life. My observation while training in France was that patients utilized Mesotherapy only when they felt they had gotten off track and gained too much weight.

Build Muscle

I love to ask my patients the following riddle: A girl graduates from high school, weighs 120 pounds, and is a size six. Five years later, she still weighs 120 pounds and went up four sizes in clothing. What happened? The answer: Her muscle converted to fat. Because muscle not only weighs more, but takes up less inches, she didn't seem to gain weight, but she did go up four sizes. This is why the scale goes up a bit when you start building muscle with anaerobic training, or lifting weights. Muscle weighs twice as much as fat, but takes up less room.

When we diet, however, we lose precious muscle. Since muscle burns calories even while sitting and sleeping, we don't want to lose an ounce of it. Those commercials telling you that you can lose ten pounds of fat per week are fooling you. You will really only lose water, and, more importantly, muscle. With each week spent immobile, you lose 0.9% of fat-burning muscle. In order to lose weight and build muscle, you must exercise.

Eat Smaller Portions More Frequently

You may not be eating frequently enough throughout the day. Rather, you may be eating the majority of your calories in one meal, and usually at night. As a result, you will have nutritional deficiencies, which then slow your metabolism leading to fat storage. Studies demonstrating that 2000 calories spread throughout the day caused weight loss, whereas 2000 calories at one meal caused weight gain. This is analogous to drinking three glasses of wine a day during meals, as the French do, spreading their calories over an entire week, versus drinking 21 glasses of wine on Saturday evening.

Get Proper Fiber

Fiber is of paramount importance. The insoluble fibers include whole grains, nuts, legumes, and some vegetables. The soluble fibers are fruits, vegetables, oats, barley, beans, and peas. Studies done with fiber demonstrated fiber alone resulted in 50 to 100 percent more weight loss than caloric restriction alone. One word of caution with fiber is to start low, and go slow. Begin with four to five grams of fiber per day and gradually raise the fiber grams. The goal is 20-40 grams of fiber per day. It is absolutely essential that you drink enough water in order to prevent constipation. Drinking insufficient amounts of water will lead to weight gain as effectively as overindulging. Water flushes toxins, and breaks down fat to be expelled.

Maintain a Healthy Liver

Many patients find weight loss is very slow or they lose weight and then plateau. They come to me with a long list of over-the-counter and physician-prescribed drugs, all of which must be processed by the liver. This only hinders their weight loss efforts. When they reduce as much medication as possible, what was once thought to be an inability to lose weight is soon remedied. This is because your liver is your major fat-burning organ.

One of my European patients came to me for weight loss. She had experienced 24 surgeries, many of which were done in Europe. It was not a big surprise that her liver enzymes were astronomically elevated from the massive amounts of anesthesia received for the surgeries, and processed through the liver. Of course, every specialist in our armamentarium was consulted to insure there was not a medical malady that could be treated with conventional allopathic medical care. This patient will not lose weight until we regenerate her liver with lipotrophics. This is the greatest strength of the liver- it is a regenerative organ, capable of repair.

The liver, when healthy, makes bile, which breaks down fat. Every day your liver produces about a quart of bile that emulsifies and absorbs fat in the small intestine. Bile cannot do its assigned task of breaking down fat if you are lacking certain nutrients, or if your liver is thickened with chemicals, toxins, excess sex hormones, heavy metals, or pharmaceuticals in excess.

What will help clean the liver? Water, water, and more water. Other lipo-throphic, or liver-cleansing, modalities include: milk thistle, pantethine, dandelion, lipoic acid or thiotic acid, phosphatidylserine, B complex vitamins, all nineteen antioxidants, garlic, onions, lecithin, broccoli, brussels sprouts, kale, gingerroot, turmeric, Oregon grape root, Myer's intravenous infusions, and inositol. I personally have periodic intravenous treatments with phosphatidylcholine in order to keep my liver enzymes in the anti-aging thirty-year old range forever. It is difficult to do everything. We simply need to educate ourselves, and pick the few that can be incorporated into our lives. It is well worth it because our heath is our greatest asset.

Eat Slowly

We are not what we eat, but what we digest. Most of us chew only about three to four times, but since chewing stimulates the satiety center of your brain, this is not nearly enough. It takes 20 minutes for the brain to acknowledge you have eaten, so if you eat too fast, your body will not have time to feel "full". You will undoubtedly feel hungry again very shortly after eating.

Eating slowly also allows the enzymes in your body to properly absorb your food. Enzymes are required to break down your food so you can get the nutrients you require. The pancreas is one organ that produces enzymes that metabolize your food. As people age, the pancreatic secretion of enzymes diminishes. Your body becomes deficient in nutrients, not to mention toxic. Digestion cannot happen without enzymes that actually activate the millions of chemical reactions that occur daily. With poor digestion, you will undoubtedly experience weight gain.

The aging of the pancreas is not the only reason for our pancreas' insufficient enzyme production. Cooked and processed foods play havoc with depleting our enzyme reserve. Raw fruits and vegetables contain enzymes. This is why it is so important to eat a salad every day. Also, heavy metals, trans fatty acids, irradiated food, microwaving, cooking at high temperatures (enzymes in foods are destroyed once heated above 118 degrees Fahrenheit), pesticides and chemicals all contribute to our pancreas' inability to secrete digestive enzymes and thereby digest our food.

Enzymes taken between meals act like hungry warriors getting rid of unwanted material, such as the waste that is produced when food breaks down. Some enzymes are given with meals to help us digest, and some are given between meals to mop up metabolic breakdown products floating around in the bloodstream.

Brown Fat

We need to learn about brown fat, which is different from the white or yellow fat we see as we make the initial incision in surgery. Babies have a lot of brown fat. Brown fat is good because it actually burns calories. White or yellow fat just sits there and doesn't require any calories to remain alive. Brown fat contains a lot of mitochondria, which generate energy through an oxidative process. Brown fat is the body's furnace, and yellow fat is the fuel. If we lose even a tiny little bit of brown fat, say one percent, it is quite easy to gain about thirty pounds of the white or yellow fat over a ten to fifteen year period. Brown fat actually generates about 25% of the heat generated in the body. We lose brown fat as we age, and as a result of exposure to environmental toxins, with fasting, crash diets, Diabetes, medications, and Hypothyroidism. To increase brown fat, we should take the essential fatty acids, particularly gamma-linolenic acid (GLA), especially if you are a Mesotherapy patient.

A good way to preserve brown fat is to start a program of GLA and MCTs that will enhance fat burning. MCTs, or medium chain triglycerides, are a form of natural fat which tends to increase your resting metabolic rate. Good sources of MCTs are grapeseed and coconut oils. There are some other herbs, amino-acids, and hormones that will help you increase thermogenesis. These include: garlic, cayenne, ginger, ginseng, Citrimax from the herbal extract Garcinia cambogia (a natural appetite suppressant), green tea, HCA (Hydroxycitric Acid), Carnitine, DHEA, melatonin, certain treatments for subclinical and clinical under-active thyroid, and Gymnena sylvestre, which, when applied to the tongue, makes sugar taste like butter. Of course, exercise will also help preserve brown fat.

Exercise

If my higher power told me I can have one of three magic bottles for healing; aspirin, cortisone, or exercise—I would choose exercise. These incredible bodies we were born with are designed for movement. As we become more and more technologically advanced, our index finger seems to be the most overworked muscle. Exercise, both aerobic and anaerobic, does well over 100 things that benefit our health now and in the future. For years, we have been jumping around doing aerobics. MRI studies at the beginning of a one year aerobic training course and one year after demonstrate that aerobic exercise may actually decrease muscle mass. This is not to say you should not do aerobic exercise; however, it is important to know that it is not as effective as anaerobic exercise, or lighting weights. If you begin weight lifting with free weights or machines, you will soon see bones and muscle you thought were gone forever.

Learn to De-Stress

There are a variety of ways to reduce and control stress levels. One study shows that Transcendental Meditation not only increases intelligence because we are quiet and listening, but it also decreases blood levels of cortisol, the stress hormone that aids in storing fat. Acupuncture is also a proven means of managing food cravings. Whichever method you choose to reduce stress, don't forget that this is an integral part of weight loss because it is both a physical and emotional process. By understanding the link between food and emotion, you will be better able to control both what and how you eat.

These are all important steps you must take to losing weight and achieving longevity. However, the most important step of all is what we will look at next: What to eat.

4

Fat Actually Helps You Lose Weight

Nearly 80 million Americans are too fat, but are deficient in essential fatty acids, also known as "the good fats". They are missing the essential fatty acids—the omega 3 and omega 6 fatty acids that our bodies are unable to synthesize. These essential fats increase your basal metabolic rate—the rate at which your body burns calories—and actually travel to a part of your brain called the ventromedial nucleus of the hypothalamus, which tells you that you are not hungry. In fact, the right fats can help you lose weight during and after Mesotherapy treatments are completed. My patients report that when they partake of enough protein and good fats, they are not hungry. Fat is the satiety nutrient so you are not hungry.

In order to understand fat after being told for decades that fat makes you fat, we need to have a brief course in Fat 101: There are different kinds of fats, and each will do something different to your body.

Saturated Fats—these are the fats that are solid at room temperature and primarily found in animal foods. Another way to get saturated fat is to eat lots of sugar, or carbohydrates. Your body produces saturated fats from sugar and this is one of the main reasons why low fat foods do not decrease body fat. A food with high sugar content is converted into stored fat in the body. These are the bad fats you should not partake on a regular basis. But the fat-phobic media left out vital information. Fat is not the enemy.

Unsaturated Fats—include the monounsaturated fats like olive oil (the greener, the better, in glass containers purchased in small amounts for purity), and the polyunsaturated fats, which contain the omega 3 and omega 6 essential fatty acids.

Hydrogenated and trans fatty acids—these are the fats you are eating when you purchase most food items that are prepackaged. The fats are hydrogenated to extend their shelf life, and to increase profit margin. If fats were not hydrogenated, the grocery store shelved food would be green and have little critters flying around the package. In other words, it would be real food. These hydrogenated/trans fatty acids get nice and homey within our cellular membranes—all 100 trillion of them, and clog our precious cellular membranes. The thousands of biochemical events that are supposed to be occurring every minute are unable to because our cells are now stiff from the hydrogenated/trans fatty acids. My patients are instructed not to eat any food that requires training in organic chemistry. In other words, they should understand what is in the ingredients label.

The Essential fatty acids—include the Omega 3 and the Omega 6 fatty acids. They are called "essential" because our bodies are unable to make them. The American diet does contain Omega 6 fatty acids because we use corn as an ingredient in many of our foods. However, Americans have a serious deficiency of Omega 3 fatty acids and require supplementation in the form of EPA/DHA (eicosahexapentanoic acid and docosahexanoic acid). The essential fatty acids are vitally important for brain and eye development, affect smooth muscle function, inflammatory processes, constrict and dilate blood vessels, and tell the ventromedial nucleus of your hypothalamus that you are not hungry. The good fats also make your stomach release CCK (Cholecystokinin), which then sends a message to your brain that you are full.

"Good fats", like the unsaturated fats and the essential fatty acids, unlock stored fat and produce satiety for up to six hours, so you don't crave carbohydrates. The good fats also slow down the release of carbohydrates, which helps regulate insulin, a fat-storing hormone. We also need the good fats to stay healthy and help us think. The brain is 60% fat, and our 100 trillion cells are encased in a fatty membranous layer which protects us against bad things like allergens, bacteria, viruses, and the like. The essential fatty acids act as an anti-inflammatory, a hormone actually, called Prostaglandin E-1 (PGE1). Essential fatty acids transmit nerve impulses and produce essential hormones that assist with thought processes.

Many of my patients ask if they should take flax oil. Flax oil is approximately 60% Omega 3 fatty acids, and 20% Omega 6 fatty acids. 12 flax oil pills are equivalent to 1 tablespoon of flax oil. They stay fresh for about three weeks in the refrigerator. Since the majority of Americans' diets already contain enough Omega 6 fatty acids, it's important to push the Omega 3 fatty acid pathway. Flax oil is a good fat, and will therefore help you lose weight, but after exposure to light and oxygen, it's not as effective. It's important to take this into consideration when deciding whether or not to take flax oil.

The best fat by far, however, is CLA, which, if you remember, is present in much of the food the French eat. It is only found in grass fed beef and dairy. It cannot be found in low-fat dairy products. CLA is good fat that helps us lose weight and remain lean. CLA also functions as an antioxidant and strengthens the immune system. It can also decrease cholesterol, decrease the amount of food that is stored as body fat, increase the amount of fat that is excreted in the feces, increase the rate at which you burn calories, control enzymes that release fat from your cells, block absorption of fat into the fat cell, decrease blood sugar, and normalize insulin levels to prevent fat accumulation. For it to do all this, you only need to take more than 1000 mg (one gram) prior to your meal.

5

What's Wrong With The Atkins Diet? : What To Eat

In order to be lean, you must eat enough protein, ensure you supplement with the good fats (notably EPA/DHA, Borage Oil, and CLA), and partake of complex carbohydrates in moderation. This sounds a lot like the Atkins Diet, and it is close; however, it requires some tweaking. The diet is totally on track in some areas, but woefully inadequate in others.

First, it is important to include complex carbohydrates, as they produce Serotonin, Dopamine, and even opiates. Without them, you will be cranky and unhappy. Complex carbohydrates are vegetables and some fruits. They contain phytochemicals that enhance our immune system. Over one hundred phytochemicals may be present in a serving of vegetables. Raw vegetables also contain enzymes and chlorophyll to alkalinize your body. Secondly, overindulgence in allowable fats will eventually harm you. The fats need to be taken in the form of good fats, not the hydrogenated, trans fatty acids that cause major chronic degenerative diseases. Simply because certain things are okay on the Atkins Diet does not mean that they are no longer dangerous. To eat a pound of bacon, four eggs, and butter and heavy cream is the same whether you are on Atkins or not.

The best way to begin your quest to lose weight and achieve longevity is to regulate what you eat. Clean out your pantry and refrigerator. Throw out everything that is not "real food"; all the junk food, low-fat food, and the food with ingredients you can't pronounce. If you don't start this way, you will only hinder yourself, as well as hurt yourself. The enrichment and processes of our food reduces its nutritional value, leaving it almost useless to our bodies.

One of the many benefits of eating real food—food that isn't processed, packaged, chemicalized and full of sugar- is that you will see your palate becomes reeducated in about three weeks. Three weeks, according to the studies, is the time it takes to develop new habit strengths. With enough protein and the good fats, to say it again, you will not be hungry, and you will be able to lose weight. Once your blood sugar is stabilized, there may even be times when there is junk food in your house and you don't hear it calling your name.

Protein is fish, meat, chicken, turkey, pork, cheese, dairy, eggs, beans and nuts. If you eat enough protein, you won't be hungry, and you won't crave sugar. Learning about what protein is, and its myriad functions, is vital for longevity. If the body is missing even one of the nine essential amino acids, your muscle will break down to get what it needs. Losing even an ounce of muscle is tragic as it lowers the rate at which you burn calories, which then causes us to burn fewer calories and store fat. You should eat protein because protein makes muscle, rebuilds immune cells, maintains fluid balance, and helps blood sugar remain stabilized, among other things.

To figure out how much protein you need in your diet, divide your weight by two and that is approximately how many grams of protein you need a day. If you weigh 160 pounds, you require 80 grams of protein a day. Meat, fish, chicken, turkey, pork that is the size of your palm is approximately 20 grams of protein. An egg is about six to eight grams of protein. Protein drinks are labeled, and I usually use two scoops, which is about 30 grams of protein. 30 grams is about the most your body can absorb in the duration of one meal.

On the Atkins diet, you get a lot of protein, but you also get a lot of toxins, unless you eat all-organic meat. These are most present in non-organic beef, which comes from caged cattle. When cattle are caged, they are stressed and produce lots of cortisol, one of the fat-storing hormones. They are also force fed, given antibiotics and given hormones and other unhealthy substances, including bovine human growth hormone, antibiotics, pesticides, insecticides, herbicides, and estrogen. Also, the method with which they slaughter the meat may nick the intestines where E. coli live, so they then irradiate the food to kill the E. coli. If you decide to go on the Atkins Diet, your intention should not be to partake this toxic load, but to become healthy and lean. While you shouldn't cut out proteins, you should supplement your diet with other types of proteins so that you can decrease the amount of toxins taken into your body.

It is best to take Whey protein shakes, where two scoops give about 32 grams of protein. You should also find a protein bar that you like, and use it for those not so infrequent times when you do not have time to stop and eat. With enough protein your immune system will work better. You will form neurotransmitters, increase your metabolism about 30 percent. If you compare proteins to carbohydrates: carbohydrates only increase your metabolism by about 4 percent. Proteins also increase the pancreatic hormone glucagon, which mobilizes fat, carries waste to the liver for detoxification, and maintains fluid balance. You won't look so puffy and your Mesotherapy treatments will produce better results. Occasionally one hears that you are getting too much protein. However, in my experience, few people eat eight pieces of chicken or salmon. Seventeen cookies, yes, this is possible, it is done, and it is fattening. To look lean, chiseled, you need protein.

Eggs are a rich source of our sulfur-based amino acids, which are another essential element in losing weight and staying healthy, as sulfur detoxifies. These sulfur-based amino acids include Taurine, Cysteine, Methionine, and Phosphytidylcholine. There are 22 amino acids, nine of which are essential, meaning our bodies are unable to make them. Vegetarians are usually deficient in essential amino acids; mainly Carnitine, Lysine, Methionine, Taurine, and Tryptophan. In my experience, vegetarians' labs show multiple deficiencies, and despite their protein-absent diets, they are still able to gain weight like the rest of us. In order to maintain a vegetarian lifestyle and still be healthy, you should combine foods to make complete proteins; like beans and rice.

My patients tell me they eat soy. Soy is a complex bean, which is very difficult to digest. Soy is also a common food allergen: many who are sensitive to milk are sensitive to soy as well. Soy contains enzymes which remove minerals like zinc and iron. Soy also lacks the essential amino acid Methionine, containing sulfur, which acts like a Pac Man detoxifier.

However, there is a healthy side to soy, but that is not what we are usually eating. The kind of soy we should be eating is cultured, fermented, unprocessed soy—namely tempeh, tofu, miso, and soy sauce. Then there is the processed soy Americans are eating, soy milk, soy peanuts, and soy protein drinks. Soy is a fine alternative to regular protein, but only when it is not processed and fermented, and only a few times a week.

As stated above, carbohydrates are fruits and vegetables, and they are not completely bad. However, it is correct that eating carbohydrates has contributed to our obesity epidemic because carbohydrates are easily attainable. When your blood sugar is low and you are hungry, you will find and eat refined carbohydrates, things like bread, pasta, donuts, pretzels, potato chips, peanut butter crackers, cookies, etc. Then your pancreas sends out lots of insulin to lower your blood sugar, which has now become too low because we just ate refined carbohydrates. The insulin has caused our blood sugar to become lower than it was before, and we are hungry again.

In order to control this process while keeping complex carbohydrates in your diet, you merely need to educate yourself on refined carbohydrates. Also remember that protein and the good fats not only keep us lean, but prevent this constant hunger thing we have.

There is not a one size fits all dietary regime, but for most people obtaining quality protein and the good fats produces lean results. My patients are instructed to listen to their own physician within. Some patients have no ill effects if they limit themselves to one junk food day per week. Others crave carbohydrates to the exclusion of all other foods if they have one M & M.

6

Drink Responsibly

Knowing what to drink in order to lose weight and feel healthy is equally as important as knowing what to eat. Certain drinks can cause just as many problems as certain foods. If you are drinking soda or fruit juice, the pancreas and stomach interpret them as a carb load, send out a lot of insulin and, store fat. Even diet soda is interpreted by your body as a sugar load and the fat storing hormone is secreted bountifully. If we want to lose weight, we must start by looking at both what we eat, and what we drink.

Soda has no nutritive value. It utilizes any minerals you may have to metabolize the 10 to 12 teaspoons of sugar it contains. Its phosphorous content leaches calcium from your bones. Then there is diet soda, which contains Aspartame or Nutrasweet. Aspartame is a neurotoxin, which means it adversely affects the brain. It converts to formaldehyde in your body. Studies have linked the sweeteners in Diet Soda to the obesity epidemic, as well as many other common ailments. If you are using artificial sweeteners, there are herbal alternatives that will help you stay healthy. May I suggest using Stevia or Stevia Plus, which is a sweet herb, good for your aging pancreas. It is available in powder and liquid forms.

Coffee is also a toxic load for our already overburdened bodies. Decaffeinated coffees are also dangerous, as they are processed with arsenic and trichlorothylene or methylchloride, chemicals also used in dry cleaning. For those who can't stop drinking coffee, organic coffee in moderation is acceptable. There is an herbal coffee available in specialty stores called Teecino. It is a very good alternative to drinking regular coffee. For decaffeinated coffee lovers, inspect the labels. Some decaf coffees are water processed and safe.

What's left? Fruit Juice. However, fruit juice, as stated above, is just as unhelpful when trying to lose weight as soda and coffee. The stomach and pancreas react to the sugars in fruit juice, increasing insulin, which lowers blood sugar, and causes us to feel hungry again. Also, when the juice is pressed, the pulp is removed, along with the vitamins and essential minerals our bodies are unable to make. When you drink a large glass of orange juice, you probably think you are getting Vitamin C. Unfortunately, much of that is lost when orange juice is exposed to oxygen and light.

Alcohol is yet another sugar. It is interpreted by the body as pure sugar. For each glass of wine, you require one glass of water, or you will become dehydrated. Once again, as with all the other drinks we have talked about, your arsenal of minerals will be required to metabolize the alcohol. If you are healthy and lean, moderate intake of wine is allowable. The French doctors delighted in teaching me that wine contains many salubrious components, including Resveratrol, proanthocyanidins, and antioxidants, to name a few. Please note that "moderate intake" are the operative words.

Besides sticking to mostly water, you may also drink Cranwater. Cranwater contains organic acids, which emulsify fat. Real 100% organic cranberry juice acts like a Sherman tank in breaking down that cottage cheese-thigh cellulite. Cranwater is the only juice I want you to drink because it cleans the lymphatic system. To prepare it, add four ounces or so of cranberry juice in twenty-eight ounces of filtered water. The label should only read: cranberry juice. No sugar, no fructose, no corn syrup; just cranberry juice. Be prepared because it is pricey, but it goes a long way.

Your main goal is to develop the habit of drinking healthy beverages like water, water with lemon, teas, and cranwater. Also, be sure to realize that transgressions are to be expected from time to time. I believe that how we nourish our bodies affects our longevity and function, but I am concerned that being hell-bent on a totally organic experience could be quite damaging to our health. Your goal is not to become a "health nut", but to learn more about what and how to eat, and attempt to make some more informed decisions concerning the food you eat.

7

What is Mesotherapy?

In the United States, thin is in, and Rubenesque is out. Having love handles, saddlebags, sausage arms, and abdominal fat is not considered attractive. If these are your concerns, Mesotherapy could become your new favorite word. We have been told that there are areas of fat in our body that are resistant to fat loss despite good nutrition and exercise. With Mesotherapy, even those areas can be reduced or even eliminated. This is known as spot fat reduction.

Dr. Michel Pistor invented Mesotherapy in 1952. Following decades of debate, Mesotherapy was being taught at the Faculty of Medicine in Paris. Mesotherapy has been done for 50 years for fat reduction and for orthopedic and rheumatologic indications. Mesotherapy done in France, Switzerland and Brazil have recently piqued our curiosity. In Europe, over 15, 000 physicians utilize Mesotherapy, and estimates indicate 60,000 people receive treatment every year. For 50 years, Europeans have been doing Mesotherapy with great results, and yet it has only come to the attention of American doctors recently. French doctors have only trained about 10 American physicians. Don't be surprised if you meet rejection when you discuss Mesotherapy with a physician who has not been trained in this European technique. As mentioned previously, the majority of doctors in the US only accept crossover-controlled double-blind studies. You must remember that the placebo effect doesn't sustain 50 years. Any therapy or treatment that's been done for 50 years has stood the test of time.

Of major interest to me was the fact that Mesotherapy has many other indications besides fat loss. It is also good to relieve migraines, herpes zoster, alopecia, poor circulation, inflammatory pathologies including back problems, microtears, lateral epicondylitis (tennis elbow), plantar fascitis, muscular spasms (including fibromyalgia) and sports injuries. Since the medication(s) are injected, they bypass the need for liver detoxification, the amount of medication is not systemically absorbed and, as a result, only 1/60 of the amount of medication normally prescribed for those ailments is required.

Before Mesotherapy, the only option in America for spot reduction was liposuction. However, liposuction is not a desirable procedure for most people. The anesthesia is difficult for some to tolerate, and the recuperation time is not possible for our baby boomers that are moving at the speed of light. Also, liposuction removes fat, but when weight is regained, the fat accumulates in areas where liposuction cannot be done, such as the midriff area. Liposuction cannot be performed on the midriff area beneath the breasts because some of your vital organs reside there. If you overeat after having this costly procedure, your tummy may remain flat, but you will develop fat in other areas.

Mesotherapy can be used to body sculpt without the need to be anesthetized. Thin patients desiring spot reduction of fat and the overweight patient requiring more guidance are both excellent candidates. My sense is that if patients start losing inches, they will be more motivated to exercise, learn about nutrition, and become lean again. Please note that Mesotherapy can be permanent if the patient practices a healthy lifestyle, but treatment for cellulite may require additional maintenance visits. The causes of cellulite, or lipodystrophy as the French call it, may be improved and corrected.

The hard and fast facts are that you are not born with a predetermined number of fat cells at birth. Fat cells increase in number during the first year of life and during puberty. Some people have fat cells, which are dispersed fairly evenly, and if they overeat and don't exercise often enough, they will become obese. Some have areas where more fat cells accumulate. You know where they are; love handles in men, saddlebags in women, and my formerly baggy knees. For 50 years we have been told we cannot spot reduce and localized fat is much more difficult to eradicate. Mesotherapy proves this is an outdated concept.

8

How does Mesotherapy Work?

What is fat?

In order to understand how Mesotherapy works, you must first understand how fat forms. Inside each fat cell, there is a gathering of fatty acids from food, chylomicrons in the intestine, and lipoproteins in the liver. This gathering has a low density- thanks to lipoprotein lipase- which transforms it into glycerol and fatty acids. In simpler terms, it turns into fat. Fat also forms via the synthesis of triglycerides, which are insulin-dependent, and derive from glucose and amino acids.

Hormones and fat are intimately related. After puberty, female fat is twice as abundant. The majority of fat is located below the waist, in the thighs, buttocks, saddlebags, and knees. Females have stored fat that is resistant to our attempts to eliminate it, insuring sustenance in the event we become with child. Too much estrogen and progesterone increases the volume of fat cells in some locations, while testosterone decreases the number and volume of fat cells.

Americans measure fat in only one way, where the French have four different ways. We simply get on the scale, which is incredibly imprecise. Since muscle weighs more than fat, you may actually gain a pound or two, but the tape measure shall tell a different story. You can lose five pounds, and when you measure yourself, realize you lost twelve inches.

The French have far more precise ways of measuring fat. They use thermography, a method that can see fat cells that have a lower temperature due to decreased oxygen supply. Secondly, they use computerized tomography (CT), which offers a number on the thickness of the fatty tissue beneath your skin, and differentiates between normal tissue and fatty tissue. People with less than 10 mm are lean, and those with more may demonstrate 50 mm of fatty tissue (about two inches). The French also use densitometry, which gives a good measurement of exactly how much fat, muscle, and bone you have in your body. Last, but not least, they also do a Doppler of the veins, which tells you the quality of blood flow. This is state of the art fat measurement, not yet done in the US. These are things the average bathroom scale cannot do.

How Does Mesotherapy Work?

Mesotherapy treatment stimulates the mesoderm, or middle layer of skin, which then aids in the process of fat loss. Small amounts of medications, vitamins, and homeopathics are injected just beneath the surface of the skin to break down fat, improve circulation, lymphatic, and venous drainage. With the addition of Vitamin C, the tone and quality of the outer layer (epidermis) of skin is improved. Microinjections are usually given twice a week over a period of four to eight weeks. In Paris, I observed different doctors putting patients on different treatment schedules. Usually, it was once a week.

The medications for Mesotherapy may contain up to 10 ccs. of solution, depending on the areas to be treated. Approximately 1 cc is injected 1 mm beneath the skin. Some physicians in the United States do an individual section. My practice does all the areas beneath the neck requiring modification. The face is done separately.

Since the medication is not injected intramuscularly, there is no systemic absorption. We have bypassed your liver, or more specifically, Phase I and Phase II detoxification of the liver. The Mesotherapy solution is comprised of various lipolytic medications to break down fat, vasodilatation medications to increase circulation, and venotonic medications to aid lymphatic drainage. Homeopathic, vitamin, and thyroid hormone may also be added.

The treatment medications fall into six categories, depending on what the patient wants to concentrate on- lipolysis, vasodilation, lymphatic drainage, circulation, edema, and skin flaccidity. Different ingredients are used for each. For lipolysis, or the breakdown of fat, Fucus Vesiculosis, Lipostabil, Yohimbine, Chophytol, Thyroxine, and Caffeine are used. For vasodilatation, Procaine, Ginkgo Biloba, Coumarin, and Pentoxifylline are used. For lymphatic drainage, the homeopathic Hammamelis is used. For circulation Torental and Fonzylane are used. For edema, Cynara Scolinum is used. And for skin flaccidity, Centelia Asiatica is used. Note that some of the ingredients mixed for the breakdown of fat include homeopathics, hormones, and medications.

Mesotherapy is done via injection inserted 2-6 mms with a very tiny needle, at an angle between 30 to 60 degrees. The maximum does of the vial cannot exceed 10 ml. Every 7-8 cm (every 3 inches) are injected with 0.05—0.1 ml of solution. Another technique is to inject every 5-10 mm at a depth of 2-4 mms. This technique is done perpendicular to the skin. Also, hematomas, or collections of blood beneath the skin's surface, are extremely rare with 2-4 mms-deep injections. A third technique is subcutaneous injections, 4-13 mms deep, in areas of intense fat accumulation, like male abdominal fat.

You can increase the area threefold if you inject a smaller amount of solution (0.005 ml) and increase the number of injections. The area is then stimulated and clears the lymphatic system. An injection in well-oxygenated skin produces a better result because it causes better absorption.

It is also important to note that the tone of the skin also influences how Meso-therapy should be approached. Darker skin tends to be more sensitive, so the thinnest needle must be used, and it is necessary to change it frequently. Typically, a test area must be done, and heparin is to be avoided as it may cause skin dyschromia or discoloration. The injection for darker skin tones should be no deeper than 3 mm.

Reducing Cellulite By Unclogging Your Lymphatic System

The mechanism by which Mesotherapy works is via the c3-5 AMP cycle, which is very complicated biochemistry. There are two types of receptors in the fat membrane. The first are adrenergic beta 1, 2 and 3, which activated adenylcyclase, an enzyme that breaks down fat. The second are alpha 2 receptors, which inhibit adenylcyclase from working. This is what makes the removal of fat very difficult. Guess where those alpha 2 receptors are? In those areas where we were previously told could not be spot reduced!

The transformation of this cAMP cycle is regulated by phosphodiesterase, which, by a feedback mechanism, slows down or stimulates the activation of the lipase responsible for hydrolysis of triglycerides. When the veins and lymphatic system are sluggish, there is an accumulation of debris, and subsequent water retention. Your lymphatic system becomes overwhelmed, and debris gets stuck. A high triglyceride number portrayed on your laboratory studies, caused mainly by overeating carbohydrates, is stored as fat. Your fat cells hypertrophy; that is to say, your fat cells are plump.

Some understanding of what a sluggish lymphatic system is needs to be explained. Your body contains 225,000 miles of arteries and veins. Additionally, there is another set of "pipes" called the lymphatic system, which carries fluids, and more specifically, wastes through your body. Think of your lymphatic system as your garbage disposal system. When it is clogged, we call that cellulite. Utilizing the correct ingredients in the Mesotherapy vial enables the physician to get your lymphatic system to flow more efficiently. This rids you of cellulite.

What You Should Know Before Your First Session

Patients undergoing Mesotherapy should not wear makeup, creams, or fragrance when they plan to have Mesotherapy sessions. It's also important for patients to mention if he or she is allergic to costume jewelry because they are then also allergic to chromium and nickel, the composition of the stainless steel needle. Patients are not to be treated during their menses. Mesotherapy should not be done on pregnant patients, or those with cardiac insufficiency or nephropathy. Patients should not be on a blood thinner, aspirin, or dipyridamole 48 hours prior to Mesotherapy because they inhibit formation of plaque, favoring hemotoma production. No bath, shower, sunbathing, or creaming 48 hours following the Mesotherapy session.

Mesotherapy is also a virtually painless procedure. During my training in Paris, the women were very comfortable during the Mesotherapy sessions. They chatted with their physicians, and spoke freely and laughed during the procedure. They tolerated it beautifully, with only the occasional ouch.

How many Mesotherapy sessions are required depends on the individual patient's situation. Usually 10 treatements are required for substantial weight loss. For those skinny-minnies who require isolated spot reduction, three Mesotherapy sessions usually do the trick. My practice treats patients once a week.

Patients commonly experience a loss of one inch off their waist. Measurable improvements are noticed via clothes, which are now loose, a more toned appearance to the skin, and actual tape measurements before and after treatment. It is not uncommon to lose an inch from the circumference of each thigh, as well as one inch from the abdomen after a few treatments.

9

My Personal Medical Philosophy

My patients often tell me that when they ask other physicians questions about methods or medicines that have not passed the rigors of double blind studies, they are met with arrogant, superficial, uninformed responses. Personally, I feel the four greatest words those of us who worked so very diligently to obtain a medical degree need to say are: "I do not know." The longer I "practice medicine", the more respect I have for what I don't know.

Being that I am formally trained in an allopathic residency in general medicine, endocrinology would not normally be one of my strengths. When I began to notice more and more of my patients were coming to me on FDA-approved hormone replacement therapy, but were still experiencing many untoward symptoms, I started referring them to endocrinologists. These endocrinologists would then just re-prescribed the same medication, usually at a higher dose. I knew that this could not be the only answer, so I decide to study endocrinology myself.

I studied in Belgium with the Hertoghe family. They have produced four generations of endocrinologists. Great-Grandpa was extracting bull testicles and inserting them into aging males in the 1910s for testosterone's life-enhancing mechanisms. Training with this family requires spending ten hours on the thyroid alone, not to mention cortisol, human growth hormone, estrone, estradiol, estriol, estrogen metabolites, progesterone, testosterone for men and women, oxytocin, melatonin, DHEA, and leptin. The education was invaluable, and it was also unavailable in the United States. I did not let that stop me. I learned endocrinology because my patients needed help, and I studied with the most highly respected endocrinologists in the world.

As I listen intently to the lengthy histories of how my patients became so unwell, I eventually figure which directions we need to go to bring them back to robust health. Even if I don't presently know the answer, with enough study, thinking, and history-taking, we achieve our goal. As a result, medicine for me is always fresh, continually new, and never boring. Patients and I work as a team, utilizing their unique biochemistry, medical history, lifestyle, and willingness to change.

I am able to do this, unlike other physicians, because I understand that medicine requires us to unlearn what we were previously taught was law. Most physicians' minds make a diagnosis 17 seconds after looking at you, and then promptly write a prescription. This is no place in medicine for those without confidence, or those with the fantasy of omnipotence. Physicians who are self-centered and feel they are omnipotent hurt people. True listening requires total concentration, and this is the greatest gift physicians can give to their patients.

Medicine in America, and the health status of Americans, is undergoing a deep change. We are caught in the eddies of mysterious change, and change frequently is terrifying. I foresee that the problem of not learning about nutrition will remedy itself because there will be a new specialty soon. We are not sure what it is going to be called; certainly not Alternative Medicine. Anti-Aging seems to be the word everyone understands, but anti- anything doesn't sit well with me. It may be called Integrative Medicine, Wholistic Medicine, Preventive Medicine, Longevity Medicine, Orthomolecular Medicine, or Functional Medicine. There was a point in medical history when we did not have a specialist for each organ system. For example, the cardiologists held meetings for years, gave examinations for certification, and with the passage of years and many, many medical conferences, the powers to be created the specialty we now know as Cardiology. The same scenario is happening with Anti-Aging medicine. There have been meetings and examinations for years, and, as we speak, some teaching hospitals are offering a Fellowship in Integrative Medicine.

This is happening because we are starting to realize that health expectancy must accompany life expectancy. Since none of us have the goal to be nursing home patients, and pain control is usually very poor in the United States, we want to do everything we possibly can to stay healthy.

Bibliography

Atkins, Robert C., M.D. *Dr. Atkins' New Diet Revolution.* Avon Books, Inc., 1999.
—. Dr. Atkins' Age-Defying Diet Revolution. St. Martin's Press, New York, 2000.

Beinfeld, Harriet, LAc., & Efrem Korngold, LAc., O.M.D. *Between Heaven and Earth: A Guide to Chinese Medicine* (New York: Ballantine, 1991), 107.

Berschauer, F., et al. "Nutritional-Physiological Effects of Dietary Fats in Rations for Growing Pigs. 4. Effects of Sunflower Oil and Coconut Oil on Protein and Fat Retention, Fatty Acid Pattern of Back Fat and Blood Parameters in Piglets." *Archive fur Tieremahrung* 34:1 (1984), 19-33.

Bland, Jeffrey, Ph.D. From an article published in *The Journal of Clinical Endocrinology and Metabolism*, vol. 56, 1993, as quoted in "Keep Your Thyroid Healthy for Peak energy," *Health and Nutrition Breakthroughs*, January 1998.
—. "What's All the Fuss About Hydrogenated Oils? *Delicious!* (January/February 1993), 44-45.
—. "Take Your Vitamins." *Delicious!* 8:7 (October 1992), 61.

Blundell, J. E. "Serotonin and Appetite." *Neuropharmacology* 23:128 (1984), 1537-1551.

Braly, James, M.D. *Dr. Braly's Food Allergy and Nutrition Revolution* (New Canaan, CT: Keats Publishing, 1992), 60.

Bucco, Gloria. "The Margarine Myth." Delicious! (January/February 1993), 103-110.

Cabot, Sandra, M.B.B.S., D.R.C.O.G. *Liver Cleansing Diet* (Paddington, New South Wales, Australia: Women's Health Advisory Service, 1996), 66-67.

Colker, M., et al. "Ephedrine, Caffeine, and Aspirin Enhance Fat Loss Under Nonexercising Conditions." *Journal of the American College of Nutrition* 16: 5 (1997), 501.

Conti, Kathy A. "Cellulite Solution." *Delicious!* (January/February 1993), 56-58.

Council on Foods and Nutrition. "A critique of low-carbohydrate ketogenic weight reduction regimens," *Journal of the American Medical Association* 224:10 (June 4, 1973), pp. 1415-1419.

Cranson, R. W. et al. "Transcendental Meditation and Improved Performance on Intelligence-Related Measures: A Longitudinal Study." *Personality and Individual Differences* 12 (1991), 1105-1116.

Crook, William G., M.D. "Thyroid and Adrenal Hormones." *The Yeast Connection and the Woman* (Jackson, TN: Professional Books, 1995), 547-557.

Daly, P. A. et al. "Ephredrine, Caffeine, and Aspirin: Safety and Efficacy for Treatment of Human Obesity." *International Journal of Obesity* 17:1 (1993), S73S78.

Decsi, Tamas, M.D., Ph.D., et al. "Obese Kids Can Lack Antioxidants." *Journal of Pediatrics* 130 (1997), 653-655.

Dillbeck, M. C. et al. "Physiological Differences between TM and Rest." *American Physiologist* 42 (1987), 879-881.

Divi, R. L., et al. "Anti-Thyroid Isoflavones From Soybean: Isolation, Characterization, and Mechanisms of Actions." *Biochemical Pharmacology* 54:10 (November 15, 1997), 1087-1096.

Dolnick, E. "Le Paradoxe Français," Hippocrates May/June 1990, pp 37-43. "Thin-jections." *Elle Magazine.* July 2003

Erasmas, Udo. *Fats That Heal, Fats That Kill* (Blaine, WA: Alive Books, 1997).

Flatt, J. P. "Body Weight, Fat Storage, and Alcohol Metabolism." *Nutrition Reviews* 50:9 (1992), 267-270.

Garfinkel, L. "Overweight and Cancer." *Annals of Internal Medicine* 103: 6 Part 2 (1985), 1034-36. F.X.

Gittleman, Ann Louise, M.S., C.N.S. *The Fat Flush Plan*. McGraw Hill, 2002.

Goldberg, Burton, et al. *Weight Loss*. Alternative Medicine.com 2000.

Golan, Ralph, M.D. *Optimal Wellness* (New York: Ballantine, 1995), 400.

Goodman, Louis S. & Alfred Gilman. *The Pharmacological Basis of Therapeutics*. 8th edition. Toronto: The Macmillan Company, 1990.

Grey, N. J. & D. M. Kipnis. "Effect of diet composition on the hyperinsulinism of obesity." *New England Journal of Medicine* 1971, p. 827.

Guyton, Arthur C. *Basic Human Physiology* (Philadelphia, PA: W. B. Saunders, 1971).

Heini, A. F., et al. "Divergent Trends in Obesity and Fat Intake Patterns: the American Paradox? *American Journal of Medicine* 102 (March 1997), 259-264.
Fumento, Michael. *The Fat of the Land* (New York: Penguin Books, 1997), 83.

Hu, F. B., M. Stampfer, & E. B. Rimm, et al. "A prospective study of egg consumption and risk of cardiovascular disease in men and women." *Journal of the American Medical Association*, 1999; 281: pp. 1387-94.

Kelly, Jill, Ph.D. "Obesity: Nondiet Approaches for What's Eating Your Patients." *Alternative and Complementary Therapies* (October 1997), 326-332.

Kendell, A. et al. "Weight Loss on a Low-Fat Diet: Consequences of the Imprecision of the Control of Food Intake in Humans." *American Journal of Clinical Nutrition* 53:5 (1991), 1124-1129.

Kirby, Jane, R.D. "Carbs vs. Protein." *Fitness* (January/February 1997), 66.
—. "Alterations in Metabolic Rate After Weight Loss in Obese Humans." *Nutrition Reviews* 43:2 (1985), 41-42.

Kuczmarski, Robert J., Dr. PH, R.D., et al. "Weight Gain on the Rise in the United States." *Journal of the American Medical Association* 272:3 (1994), 205-211.

Langer, Stephen E. and James F. Scheer. *Solved: The Riddle of Illness* (New Canaan, CT: Keats Publishing, 1995), 31, 67.

Coz, J. Le, et al. *Mésothérapie et médicine esthétique.*

Lee, John R., M.D. *What Your Doctor May Not Tell You About Menopause—The Breakthrough Book on Natural Progesterone.* (Warner Books, 1996), pp212, 294, 297.

Lee; Lita, Ph.D., Lisa Turner, & Burton Goldberg. *The Enzyme Cure* (Tiburon, CA: Future Medicine Publishing, 1998) 25-27.
—. "Hypothyroidism: A Modern Epidemic." *Earthletter* (Spring 1994), 2.

Liscum and N. K. Dahl. "Intracellular Cholesterol Transport." *Journal of Lipid Research* 33 (1992), 1239-1254.

Livero, Peggy. "Obesity: The Next Generation." *Nourish* (February/March 1996), 8.

Ludwig, David L., M.D., Ph.D., et al. "Dietary Fiber, Weight Gain, and Cardiovascular Disease Risk Factors in Young Adults" *Journal of the American Medical Association* 282:16 (1999), 1539-1546.

Manson, J. E. et al. "Body Weight and Mortality Among Women." *New England Journal of Medicine* 333:11 (1995), 677-685.

Marin, P., M. Krotkiewski, P. Bjorntorp. "Androgen Treatment of Middle-Aged Obese Men: Effects on Metabolism, Muscle and Adipose Tissues." *European Journal of Medicine* 1: 6 (1992), 329-336.

Martineau, J. et al. "Vitamin B6, Magnesium, and Combined B-6 Magnesium: Therapeutic Effects in Childhood Autism." *Biological Psychiatry* 20 (1985), 467-468.

McMichael-Phillips, D. F., C. Harding, M. Marton, et al. "Effects of soy-protein supplementation on epithelial proliferations in the histologically normal human breast," *Am. Jrnl. of Clin. Nutr.* 11/98: 68 (6 suppl): 1431S-1435S.

Meikle, A. W. et al. "Effects of a Fat-Containing Meal on Sex Hormones in Men." *Metabolism* 39-9 (1990), 943-946.

Mowrey, Daniel B., Ph.D. "The Major Scientific Breakthrough of the 90s: Reducing Body Fat Through Thermogenics." *Health Store* news 11:5 (October/November 1994).
—. "Thermogenesis: The Whole Story." *Let's Live* (November 1995), 61-93.
—. *Fat Management: The Thermogenic Factor* (Lehi, UT: Victory Publications 1994) 17.

Muller, W. A., et al. "The influence of the antecedent diet upon glucagon and insulin secretion." *New England Journal of Medicine* 285 (1971), pp. 1450-1454

Murray, Michael, N.D. "The Importance of Dietary Fiber." *Phyto-Pharmica Review* 4:1 (1990), 1-4.

Nomura, F. et al. "Liver Function in Moderate Obesity-Study in 534 Moderately Obese Subjects Among 4,613 Male Company Employees." *International Journal of Obesity* 10 (1986), 349-354.

Olesen, E. S., F. Quaade. "Fatty foods and obesity," *Lancet* 1 (1960), pp. 1048-1051.

Xavier Pi-Sunyer, F., M.D. "The Fattening of Americans." *Journal of the American Medical Association* 272:3 (1994), 238.
—. "Health Implications of Obesity." *American Journal of Clinical Nutrition* 53:6 Suppl (1991), 1595S-1603S.

Porte, D., Jr. & S. C. Woods. "Regulation of Food Intake and Body Weight by Insulin" *Diabetologia* 20 Suppl. (March 1981) 274-280.
Moss, Jeffrey, D.D.S., C.N.S., C.C.N. "Hyperinsulinemia and Insulin Resistance-A Missing Link in Obesity and Cardiovascular Disease." *Townsend Letter for Doctors and Patients* (April 1996), 87-91.

Pouls, Maile, Ph.D. "Digestive Problems." *Alternative Medicine Digest* 18 (May/June 1997), 40.

Randolph, Theron. *An Alternative Approach to Allergies* (New York: Harper Collins, 1989).

Reid, Daniel. *The Complete Book of Chinese Health and Healing* (Boston: Shambhala, 1994), 78.

Rexrode, K. M., et al. "A Prospective Study of Body Mass Index and Risk of Stroke in Women." *Journal of the American Medical Association* 277:19 (1997), 1539-1545.

Robinovitz, Karen. "The New Lipo—Does It Really Melt Away Your Fat? *Harper's Bazaar*, October, 2002.

Rothman, K. J., et al. "Teratogenecity of High Vitamin A Intake." *New England Journal of Medicine*. 333 (1995), 1369-1373.

Rudin, D., M.D., & Clara Felix. *Omega-3 Oils: A Practical Guide* (Garden City, NY: Avery, 1996), p. 22.

Schwartz, Arthur, M.D., & M.P. Cleary. "The Effect of Dehydroepiandosterone on Body Weight Gain." *Journal of Nutrition* 117: 2 (February 1987) 406-407.

Schutz, Y. et al. "Failure of Dietary Fat to Promote Fat Oxidation: A Factor Favoring the Development of Obesity." *American Journal of Clinical Nutrition* 50:2 (1989), 307-314.

Shields, J. W., M.D. "Lymph, Lymph Glands, and Homeostasis." *Lymphology* 25: 4 (December 1992), 147-153.

Shippen, Eugene, M.D., & William Fryer. *The Testosterone Syndrome* (New York: M. Evans, 1998), 91.

Schmidt, Michael A., D.C., C.N.S., & Jeffrey Bland, Ph.D. "Thyroid Gland as Sentinel: Interface Between Internal and External Environment." *Alternative Therapies* 3:1 (January 1997), 78-81.

Sears, Barry, PhD. *The Zone* (New York: HarperCollins, 1995), 30.

Simontacchi, Carol, C.C.N., M.S. *Your Fat Is Not Your Fault* (New York: P. Tarcher/Putnam, 1997), 32.
—. "Controlling Weight No Longer Considered Dieting." *Calorie control Council press release* (May 11, 1998).
—. "New Strategies to Achieve Your Healthiest Weight: Health After 50." *Johns Hopkins Medical Letter* 7:1 (1995), 4.

Solomon, S. J., & J. D. King. "Effect of low zinc intake on carbohydrate and fat metabolism in men" *Federal Proc* 42 (1983), p. 391.

Tauber, Gary. "What If Fat Doesn't Make You Fat?" *New York Times Magazine,* July 7, 2002.

Tips, Jack, N.D., Ph.D. *Our Liver...Your Lifeline* (Ogden, UT Apple-A-Day Press, 1995), 90.

Trowell, H., Burkit, & K. Heaton. *Dietary Fiber, Fiber-Depleted Foods and Disease* (New York: Academic, 1985).

Valentine, Tom. "If You Eat Soy, Watch Your Thyroid Function: New Study." *True Health* (Autumn 1997), 1-3.

Italliem, T. Van. "Health Implications of Overweight and Obesity in the United States." *Annals of Internal Medicine* 103: 6 Part 2 (1985), 198-88.

Vettor, R., G. DoPergda, & C. Pagano, et al. "Gender differences in serum leptin in obese people: relationships with testosterone body fat distribution and insulin sensitivity." *European Journal of Clinical Investigation,* 1997 Dec: 27(2): 1016-24.

Walford, R. L., et al. "The Calorically Restricted Low-Fat Nutrient-Dense Diet in Biosphere 2 Significantly Lowers Blood Glucose, Total Leukocyte Count, Cholesterol, and Blood Pressure in Humans." *Proceedings of the National Academy of Sciences* 89:23 (1992), 11533-11537.

Walford, R. L., & M. Crew. "How Dietary Restriction Retards Aging: An Integrative Hypothesis." *Growth, Development, and Aging* 53:4 (1989 (, 139-140.

Wallace, R. K., et al. "Physiological Effects of Transcendental Meditation." *Science* 167 (1970), 1751-1754.

Ward, Carol J. G. "Weighty Resolution: Beward of Fad Dieting" *The Arizona Republic* (January 4, 1999), D3.

Waterhouse, Debra. *Outsmarting the Midlife Fat Cell* (New York: Hyperion, 1998), pp. 18-19.

Webber, E. M. "Psychological Characteristics of Bingeing and Nonbingeing Obese Women." *Journal of Psychology* 128:3 (1994), 339-351.

Widener, Andrea. "Study Warns of Danger in Meat" *Contra Costa Times.* Oct. 31, 1998.

Willett, W., et al. "Is Dietary Fat a Major Determinant of Body Fat?" *American Journal of Clinical Nutrition* 1998: 67: 556S-562S.
—. "Letter to David Kessler, M.D., Commissioner, U.S. Food and Drug Administration" (November 23, 1995).

Wright, Jonathan, M.D. *Natural Hormone Replacement for Women Over 45* (Smart Publications, 1997), p. 56.

Yanick, Paul, Jr. Ph.D. "The Amazing Chemical Plant of Our Bodies: The Liver." *Let's Live* (August 1987), 59.

Yazbech, J., et al. "Effects of Essential Fatty Acid Deficiency on Brown Adipose Tissue Activity in Rats Maintained at Thermal Neutrality." *Comparative Biochemistry and Physiology A: Comparative Physiology* 94:2 (1989), 273-276.

Yudkin, J. & M. Carey. "The treatment of obesity by the high fat diet. The inevitability of calories." *Lancet* 2 (1960), pp. 939-941.

Zhenping, Lei. "Treatment of 42 Cases of Obesity With Acupuncture." *Journal of Traditional Chinese Medicine* 8:2 (June 1988), 125-126.

Ziovdron, C. R., Strearly, & W. Klee. "Opiate peptides derived from food proteins: The exorphins," *Journal of Biochemistry.* 1979: 254:2379-2380; cited by Garrison, p. 625.
—. "Endomysium antibodies in blood donors predicts a high prevalence of celiac disease in the USA"., April 1996.

0-595-32229-8

Made in the USA
Lexington, KY
16 September 2011